EAT SMART, NOT LESS

Take Control of Your Life and Lose Weight the Healthy Way

By

K. CONNORS

© **Copyright 2017 By K. Connors - All Rights Reserved.**

Copyright © 2017 *Eat Smart, Not Less*. All rights reserved. No part of this publication may be reproduced, distributed, or transmitted in any form or by any means, including photocopying, recording, or other electronic or mechanical methods, without the prior written permission of the publisher, except in the case of brief quotations embodied in critical reviews and certain other noncommercial uses permitted by copyright law. This also includes conveying via e-mail without permission in writing from the publisher. All information within this book is of relevant content and written solely for motivation and direction. No guarantees. All information is considered valid and factual to the writer's knowledge. The author is not associated or affiliated with any company or brand mentioned in the book, therefore does not purposefully advertise nor receives payment for doing so.

Table of Contents

Introduction: Why You Should Eat Smarter and Not Less 1

The Health Benefits 3

Motivation and Motivating Factors 5

Setting Goals For Weight Loss 7

Tracking Your Results... 9

Dieting: The Art of Calorie Management 13

Juicing Recipes 16

How To Fight Cravings 22

The Importance of Cardio Workouts... 30

How to Keep The Weight Off After Losing It 33

Myths About Dieting and Workouts... 36

Introduction: Why You Should Eat Smarter and Not Less

Can you weigh less without eating less? Have you tried to lose weight by cutting down the amount of food you eat? Do you end up feeling hungry and not satisfied? Or have you avoided trying to lose weight because you're afraid of feeling hungry all the time? If so, you are not alone.

Contrary to popular belief, you don't have to starve yourself to death to lose weight; one can eat more frequently and actually lose weight. It's just the smarter and healthier way. There is so much emphasis these days on finding that perfect diet or ideal meal replacement or just simply curbing those food cravings when there should be much more on educating ourselves on proper nutrition.

Meal replacements and protein shakes can play an important role in our diets, but they are not made for us to live on alone. Sure, it would be easier if we could just find that magic formula out there and not have to worry about food and know that we are doing the best for our bodies; however, there's none, as of yet. Besides, what fun would that be for our taste buds?

Many people throw in the towel on weight loss because they feel deprived and hungry when they eat less. Have no fear, there is another way. Aim for slow, steady weight loss by decreasing calorie intake while maintaining an adequate nutrient intake and increasing physical activity. You can cut calories by eating more nutritious food. The key is to eat foods that will fill you up without consuming plenty of calories. If I cut calories, won't I be hungry? Nope! Research shows that people get full by the amount of food they eat, not the number of calories they take in. You can cut calories in your favorite foods by lowering the amount of fat and/or increasing the number of fiber-¬rich ingredients, such as vegetables or fruit.

A healthy diet doesn't mean you have to starve; however, for many, they think it does. By depriving your body of the essential nutrients that food supplies us with, you are, without a doubt, hurting that body you have worked so hard get. Without food, you may soon find yourself lacking energy, concentration, focus, and desire. Not to mention developing what could become a serious health issue. Of course, exercise, activities, and genetics also play an important role, but eating properly and smarter are crucial to weight control, keeping energy levels up, and overall health.

Knowing what you will be eating from the moment you get up until you go to bed can make all the difference in a successful day or a not-so-successful day. Like everything in life, simple planning can bring you out of the doldrums and get you back on the right track, eating delicious food that you never thought possible!

Eat more, not less, of the right food and be sure to drink plenty of water. Combine that with the proper exercise program and you are sure to see and, more importantly, feel the desired results.

The Health Benefits

Giving your body the right type of food is paramount to your overall health. Healthy eating is not about sticking to strict nutrition facts or depriving yourself completely from the food you love. Rather, it is about feeling mentally and physically great and having good energy levels, all of which can be achieved by learning nutrition basics and making better food choices. The benefits of eating healthy by making just a few changes are exceptional. Apart from maintaining healthy and functioning organs in your body, healthy eating provides a wide array of benefits.

Less Illness and More Health

As the saying goes: You are what you eat, and you become what you eat; whatever we eat reflects on our body. Unhealthy processed and fast foods affect the normal functioning of our body systems and can lead to obesity and illness. Eating healthy provides all the required nutrients for the body, which helps in proper functioning of our body organs. By improving body functions, you are enhancing your immune system, which further helps in protecting against many chronic illnesses. Staying active and energetic is part of a good diet that is the key to a healthy body. Eating a well-balanced diet provides good nutrition and energy to continue the healthy function of the body. This also helps support healthy growth and development. When the energy requirements of the body are balanced, you stay active and energetic throughout the day.

Weight Control is Best Through Your Diet

It is no secret that exercise and a healthy diet are the keys to losing weight and maintaining it. Exercise and continuing with the wrong food will not bring your weight down, although exercise has many other health benefits and is an important part of a healthy lifestyle. A recent study has shown that half an hour of exercise will improve the brains "Plasticity." Plasticity in the brain is important for learning, memory, and motor skill conditions. This also strengthens connections between other cells and as well different brain cells. Weight loss is all about making the right food choices that will help you in losing weight and calories. Optimal body weight keeps you fit and healthy and prevents you from many obesity-related diseases.

Look Good and Feel Good

In today's lifestyle, where people are overtly conscious of their appearance, excessive weight may affect your overall looks, as perceived by others. Hence, weight control is one of the most important benefits of eating a healthy diet. Overeating and eating junk food will not only pack on the pounds, it also disturbs your sleeping patterns. On the other hand, a good diet can do just the opposite; healthy food reduces stress and helps in getting a good night's sleep. A restful sleep keeps your mind as well as body active to face the next day with a better attitude.

Motivation and Motivating Factors

Finding motivation during the process of weight loss can become very difficult. If you're like most people, you've been on a million different weight loss diets. You voraciously read magazines for their weight loss tips and gravitate toward the headlines that promise you can lose weight fast. The chances are good that you have indeed lost weight on many of these diets, but the chances are even better that you've gained it all back—plus some.

Weight Loss Diet Failure

You've probably bought into the propaganda that says you've failed at dieting; a different and more accurateway of looking at it is that the weight loss diet has failed you. This is because most diets focus on short-term changes that result in temporary weight loss, but never tackle the underlying factors that make you put on the pounds to begin with. In other words, they focus only on the "outside" problem—your body—and neglect everything below the surface—your emotions, your intellect, and your relationships. A diet for summer might work but you can bet by winter it will be back to haunt you again.

Turning Failure into Success

In order to lose weight and keep it off, you need a guide who will lead you on an exploratory journey to discover the power and control that you possess. Then, you need to be taught how to harness those powers to achieve all that you want in life—including fitting into your jeans again. You may have been told—either verbally or through insidious advertisements—that if you don't have control over your eating, you have no control at all. Nothing could be further from the truth. Every person is magnificent, and every person has mental power, emotional power, social power and physical power just waiting to be tapped into. When you heal your past wounds and recognize and reinforce the power within you, you have laid the foundation for permanent weight loss.

Practical and Fun

If a weight loss diet is a drag, you'll never succeed in reaching your goals. On the other hand, if you have an empowering program to follow that is also practical and fun, you hold the keys to success. In fact, you can even drop a whole size in two weeks. The "secret"—if you want to call it that—is to adopt a well-tested exercise program that can instantly fit into your lifestyle. Remember, the success lies in simplicity, clarity, and practicality. Then, you need to adopt an eating plan that works synergistically with your exercise plan to build on the foundation of the inner work you have done in order to embrace your personal power. Remember, with the right guide, you can do more than just getting on yet another weight loss diet; you can truly win in all areas of your life and achieve an outer beauty that matches your inner beauty.

Setting Goals For Weight Loss

If you really want to drop some pounds from your body, you need to set some goals that are practical and realistic. You should also make sure that you're making real changes to your lifestyle and eating habits.

However, don't go for a fad diet or weight loss program that promises fast and easy weight loss. There is no shortcut for losing weight. Accept the *reality*, and it will be much easier for you to take the next step.

Make a Commitment

You must have a rock-solid determination and firm commitment in order to achieve your weight loss goals. Ask yourself, do you really want to drop those extra pounds?

If *yes*, then make a commitment that you're ready to face any challenges, and no matter what happens you'll stick with your objectives. Your weight loss goals may have an impact on your lifestyle and relationship with others. So, think about that as well. Also, make some alternative plans to deal with other stresses of your life.

Set Some Small Realistic Goals

To reach your weight loss goals, you need to make at least a six-month or one-year long-term plan. It would be unrealistic to assume that you could lose 10-12 pounds per week.

Start with some small daily goals and increase those gradually. Think about something that is possible for you with minimal effort.

You can start by increasing your regular physical activity. For example, you can plan to walk for 20 minutes today or do the household work for tomorrow.

Set Some Weekly Weight Loss Goals

Think about some weekly goals that are practical and possible. I believe planning to lose 1-2 pounds (0.5 – 1 kg) per week is a realistic and attainable goal. Mathematically, one pound (0.5 kg) of fat is equal to 3,500 calories. So, to drop a pound of fat per week, you need to burn at least 3,500 calories. It means (500 calories x 7 days = 3,500 calories) you have to burn at least 500 more calories per day than you consume.

No doubt, this is an achievable target, as you only require either decreasing calorie intake or increasing physical activity to reach the calorie-burning goal.

Adopt a Healthy Eating Style

Burn more calories than you consume—the simple formula you should remember in order to lose weight. However, to lose more calories, don't go for extreme ways like fasting, water diet, or lemon juice diet. For successful, long-term benefits, you must choose a weight loss plan that follows a healthy, calorie-controlled diet combined with exercise.

Carefully prepare a diet plan, and change your eating style gradually. Make sure your body consumes adequate calories according to your height and weight. Include vegetables and fruits as a primary source of calories. Divide your calorie intake into 5-6 meals. Try replacing 3-4 meals with light foods, such as juices, snacks, fruit blends, or soups, so that you can stop unwanted hunger.

Say no to fast foods and junk foods, as they contain little or no nutritious value and are high in fat, sugar, salt, and calories. Also, you need to know that these foods are considered one of the major causes for overweight. Junk foods often contain a high amount of saturated fats that are unnatural and very difficult to absorb or digest properly. As a result, these fats remain in the body and increase extra weight.

Tracking Your Results

Scale weight can be a useful number to know but, even better, is knowing your body fat percentage. This is important because scale weight doesn't always tell the whole story. Knowing your body fat percentage can give you a better idea of how much fat you really need to lose and, even better, whether you're making progress in your program - things your scale can't tell you.

It's possible for your scale weight to remain the same, even as you slim down, especially if you're losing fat and gaining muscle.

A healthy body fat range is 25 - 31% for women and 18 - 25% for men. Get the most out of your body fat measurement by:

- Checking it once a week or every other week instead of daily. Body fat doesn't vanish overnight and you may not see those small changes if you measure every day.

- Having the same person measure you each time. Different trainers will measure you in different ways, so stick with the same person each time and make sure the person is very experienced in measuring body fat. This can also be done on your own.

- If using a bioelectrical impedance scale, be sure to measure under the same circumstances each time. Hydration, food intake, and skin temperature can affect body fat measurements.

- Keep track of your numbers in a journal or calendar.

The Right Way to Use the Scale

As mentioned, scales don't always give you the whole story about your body or your weight loss progress. For that reason, scales (when used alone) aren't the best way to track what's really going on inside your body.

Another reason to not rely solely on scales is the emotional nature of weighing ourselves. Stepping on a scale doesn't just give us a number; it can determine how we feel about ourselves and affect body image. The problem with body weight scales is that they measure everything--fat, muscle, bones, organs and even that sip of water or bite of food you've had. The scale can't tell you what you've lost or gained, which is important information if you're trying to lose weight, and by weight, what we really mean is fat.

That doesn't mean the scale is useless. In fact, it's a wonderful tool when you combine it with your body fat percentage. Knowing both of these numbers will tell you whether you're losing the right kind of weight... fat.

Simply multiply your weight by your body fat percentage. For example, a person who weighs 150 lbs. with 21% body fat has 31 lbs. of fat and 118 lbs. of lean tissue (150 x .21 = 31.5 lbs. of fat, 150 - 31.5 = 118 lean tissue).

Keeping track of these numbers on a weekly or monthly basis will help you see what you're losing and/or what you're gaining.

Try these tricks to make weighing yourself a useful and more positive experience:

- Weigh yourself first thing in the morning before you eat or drink anything.

- Weigh yourself once a month instead of daily or weekly to give your body time to respond to your weight loss program. The scale won't reflect small changes happening in your body composition.

- Remember, the scale weighs everything. Just because your scale weight hasn't changed doesn't mean you aren't making progress.

- Use scale weight along with body fat percentage for a more accurate view of your progress.

If the scale freaks you out and body fat testing isn't an option, your next best choice is taking your measurements.

Take Your Measurements

This is a great option for tracking progress because it doesn't require any fancy equipment and anyone can do it. Taking your measurements at certain areas can give you an idea of where you're losing fat, which is important since we all lose fat in different areas and in a different order.

Taking your measurements can help reassure you that things are happening—even if you're not losing fat exactly where you want just yet.

Start by wearing tight fitting clothing (or no clothing) and make a note of what you're wearing so you know to wear the same clothes the next time you measure. Here's how to do it:

- Bust: Measure around the chest right at the nipple line, but don't pull the tape too tight.

- Chest: Measure just under your bust.

- Waist: Measure a half-inch above your belly button or at the smallest part of your waist.

- Hips: Place the tape measure around the biggest part of your hips.

- Thighs: Measure around the biggest part of each thigh.

- Calves: Measure around the largest part of each calf.

- Upper arm: Measure around the largest part of each arm above the elbow.

- Forearm: Measure around the largest part of the arm below the elbow.

You can use this Progress Chart to record your measurements. Take them again once a week or once a month to see if you're losing inches.

Use Your Clothes

It may seem obvious, but don't overlook one of the simplest ways to track progress--how your clothes fit.

You may want to take a picture of yourself wearing a bathing suit and keep it in your weight loss journal. Each month, take a new picture... you'll be surprised at how many changes you notice in a picture as opposed to just seeing yourself in the mirror.

You can also use your clothes to keep track of your progress. Choose one pair of pants that are a little tight and try them on every four weeks to see how they fit. Make a note of where they feel loose, where they feel tight and how you feel wearing them.

Whatever the scale may say, your pants will never lie. Whichever method you choose to track your progress, be patient with yourself. It takes months for many of us to see significant changes and, even then, you'll probably notice the weight fluctuating as your eating habits and workouts change. The key is to stay consistent!

Dieting: The Art of Calorie Management

The number of calories in a particular amount or weight of food is called "calorie density" or "energy density." Low-calorie foods are ones that don't pack a lot of calories into each bite. Foods that have a lot of water or fiber and little fat are usually low in calorie density. They will help you feel full without an unnecessary amount of calories.

A healthy eating plan is one that:

- Emphasizes fruits, vegetables, whole grains, and fat-free or low-fat milk and milk products.

- Includes lean meats, poultry, fish, beans, eggs, and nuts.

- Is low in saturated fats, trans-fats, cholesterol, salt (sodium), and added sugars.

- Stays within your caloric needs

Let's take macaroni and cheese as an example. The original recipe uses whole milk, butter, and full-fat cheese. This recipe has about 540 calories in one serving (1 cup). However, we can use 8 ounces light cream cheese instead of 21/4 cups full-fat cheddar cheese.

Here's how to remake this recipe:

- Use 2 cups non-fat milk instead of 2 cups whole milk.

- Use 1 tablespoon of butter instead of 2 or use 2 tablespoons of soft trans--fat free margarine.

- Add about 2 cups of fresh spinach and 1 cup diced tomatoes (or any other veggie you like).

Your redesigned mac and cheese now has 315 calories in one

serving (1 cup). You can eat the same amount of mac and cheese with 225 fewer calories.

In order to be able to cut calories without eating less and feeling hungry, you need to replace some higher calorie foods with foods that are lower in calories and fat, while still filling you up. In general, this means foods with lots of water and fiber in them.

What Foods Will Fill Me Up?

To make smart food choices that are part of a healthy eating plan, you need the foods that will fill you up with fewer calories.

- Fruits and vegetables (prepared without added fat). Spinach, broccoli, tomato, carrots, watermelon, berries, apples

- Low-fat and fat-free milk products. Low or fat-free milk, low or fat-free yogurt, low- or fat-free cottage cheese

- Broth-based soup. Vegetable-based soups, soups with chicken or beef broth, tomato soups (without cream)

- Whole grains. Brown rice, whole-wheat bread, whole-wheat pasta, popcorn

- Legumes (beans and peas). Black, red kidney and pinto beans (without added fat), green peas, black-eyed peas

- Lean meat, poultry, and fish. Grilled salmon, chicken breast without skin, ground beef (lean or extra lean)

- These foods can pack more calories into each bite. Choose them less often:

- Fried foods. Eggs fried in butter, fried vegetables, french fries, fatty cuts of meat, bacon, brisket, ground beef (regular), full-fat milk products, full-fat cheese, full-fat ice cream, whole and 2% milk

- Dry snack foods. Crackers or pretzels, cookies, chips, dried fruits

- High-fat and high-sugar foods. Croissants, margarine, shortening and butter, doughnuts, candy bars, cakes and pastries

Good things can come in big packages

People eat more than they realize when faced with large portion sizes. This usually means eating too many calories. But, not all large portions are created equal. Larger portions of water and fiber-rich foods, like fruits, vegetables, and broth-based soups, can fill you up with fewer calories.

Start with an appetizer

Research shows that if you eat a low-calorie appetizer before a meal, you will eat fewer total calories during the meal. Start your meals with a broth-based soup or a green salad without a large amount of cheese, or croutons.

Fruits and veggies: Keep it simple

Most fruits and veggies are low-calorie and will fill you up, but the way you prepare them can change that. Breading and frying, and using high-fat creams or butter with vegetables and fruit will add extra calories. Try steaming vegetables and using spices and low-fat sauces for flavor and enjoy the natural sweetness of fresh fruit.

What about beverages? While drinking beverages is important to good health, they don't help you feel full and satisfied the way food does. Choose drinks without calories, like water, sparkling water, or unsweetened iced tea. Drink fat-free or low-fat milk instead of 2% or whole milk.

Juicing Recipes

Juicing on an occasional basis while gorging on unhealthy foods and living a sedentary lifestyle will not help in losing weight. It is a healthy habit that must be included in daily life to enjoy its health benefits. Consuming natural fruit and vegetable juices is extremely beneficial for detoxifying the body and is one of the best natural ways to lose weight by jump-starting the process of fat burning.

Why Should I Juice?

Well, the most common question that circles the health and fitness circle concerning juicing is whether it is better to have fruits and vegetable juice or have them whole. Having the whole fruits and vegetables is the best option indeed but there are certain reasons why juicing wins the day.

- Juicing increases overall fruit and vegetable intake, which is not possible if we are consuming them whole.

- Juicing promotes weight loss by boosting metabolism.

- Certain vegetable juices help in improving cardiovascular health and lower the level of cholesterol in the blood.

- The high content of antioxidants and fiber helps in reducing the risk of all kinds of cancer.

Although pills and crash diets are widely available and promote weight loss (supposedly), most of them have been shown to have severe side effects in the long run. Therefore, it is best to resort to natural remedies that are time tested and have no harmful effects on health. After all, isn't it our goal to become *healthier*?

Carrot and Grapefruit Smoothie

The importance of carrot juice for weight loss is well known. Carrots are extremely low in calories and high in fiber which makes carrot juice a perfect vegetable juice for weight loss. Being rich in fibers, it helps keep the tummy satiated for a longer time and prevents mindless cravings, which is one of the main reasons for weight gain. Studies show that eating grapefruit after consuming a meal high in fats can help in cutting out the calories by a fifth. Therefore, a combination of these two superfoods for weight loss makes the ideal smoothie for burning calories.

Ingredients:

- Pink Grapefruit – 1
- Carrots – 4
- Lemon Juice – 2 Tablespoons
- Ginger – 1 Inch

Peel the grapefruit and cut the inside into rough cubes. Peel and cut the carrots into small cubes. Add all the ingredients in a food processor; add the lemon juice and peeled ginger to it. Mix it for 3 to 4 minutes and pour into a tall smoothie glass and enjoy. This is one of the best home remedies for weight loss that shows great effectiveness when drank once on a daily basis.

Cucumber and Kiwi Smoothie

Cucumber is an amazing vegetable that helps to lose weight naturally, and a healthy diet for weight loss almost always includes this delicious vegetable. Being rich in water and low in sodium, it helps in reducing bloating and water retention. Comprising of mere 45 calories, it makes a surprisingly low-calorie snack that you can munch any time and also works in bulking up your salads. Kiwi fruits are loaded with energy, nutrients, and vitamins and are low in calories that make it a perfect delicious tart snack for those trying to lose weight. Kiwi is also rich in dietary fibers that help in keeping you satiated for longer, thereby preventing mindless munching.

Ingredients:

- Kiwi – 2
- Cucumber – 1
- Lime – 1/2
- Mint Leaves – A few

Peel and chop the kiwi and cucumber, put it in the blender, add a dash of lime and the mint leaves; blend well and experience the fat fighting power of this mean green smoothie.

Bell pepper and Apple Smoothie

Natural weight loss remedies must include bell peppers. The brightly colored peppers, especially the red ones are rich in capsaicin that provides it with the spicy and burning feature. Capsaicin increases body temperature and speeds up metabolism through thermogenesis that helps the body in burning calories and improving fat oxidation. Eating at least 6 mg of capsaicin on a daily basis increases the burning of abdominal fat in both men and women. Apples are low in fat, calories and sodium, and high in fibers and vitamins that make it the perfect natural weight loss food. The water soluble fibers in apples help in extracting cholesterol from the blood stream keeping the heart healthy.

Ingredients:

- Red Bell Pepper – 1
- Red Apple – 1
- Lemon Juice – 1 Tablespoon

Chop the bell pepper and the apple and add it in a blender, add the lemon juice and blend all the ingredients with 1/2 cup water for a few minutes; pour the contents into a glass, and enjoy the spicy and hot taste of this delightful red smoothie.

Celery, Cucumber and Apple Smoothie

A balanced diet for weight loss must include raw celery as a crunchy and satiating snack that doesn't add excess calories to the body. Being extremely low in calories and high in vitamins C, K, folate, potassium and dietary fibers, it also makes an important ingredient for juice diets during weight loss. A combination of celery with juicy cucumber and delicious apples help in enhancing its effectiveness for weight loss even further.

Ingredients:

- Celery Stalks – 3
- Cucumber – 1
- Red Apple – 1

Chop the celery stalks into medium sized pieces, chop the cucumber and apple and add all the ingredients in a food processor, add ½ cup of water to it and blend well to form a smooth paste. Pour into a drinking mug and enjoy with a dash of lemon.

Cucumber and Pineapple Smoothie

Pineapple, the delicious tropical fruit with refreshing flavor is useful for weight loss because of its high water and fiber content that aids in achieving your weight loss goals by keeping you satiated for longer. It also helps in suppressing appetite and reducing the craving for unhealthy snacks. Spinach and other leafy green vegetable help in preventing food cravings and are an important part of low-calorie meals such as the GM Diet and 1200 Calorie Diet plan because you can eat a lot of it without thinking about piling up calories.

Ingredients:

- Cucumber – 1
- Pineapple – 1 Cup (Chopped)
- Spinach – 1 Cup

Chop the cucumber and spinach roughly and add all the ingredients in a food processor; add ½ cup of water to it. Blend well and pour into a serving glass and enjoy the tangy and flavorful taste of this weight loss smoothie.

Tomato, Carrots and Asparagus Smoothie

The best juices for weight loss must include tomatoes. These delicious and juicy red fruits are rich in antioxidants that help in reducing the harmful effects of inflammation and fluid retention in the body. It also helps in reversing leptin resistance in the body that helps regulate metabolism, appetite and the fat burning process of the body. There are various ways in which asparagus helps in losing weight. Being a great source of soluble fibers, it helps in keeping you full, while suppressing hunger. It helps in controlling blood sugar by supporting blood glucose metabolization. It is a natural diuretic that helps in flushing out excess fluid from the body and is a natural remedy for bloating.

Ingredients:

- Tomatoes – 3 Medium Sized
- Asparagus – 6 Stalks
- Carrots – 3

Wash and chop all the vegetables roughly and add it to the food processor; add 1/4th cup of water, blend well and pour into a serving glass. Enjoy with a hint of lemon juice and mint.

How To Fight Cravings

Almost everyone experiences food cravings from time to time. For dieters, food cravings can be an unhelpful distraction and temporarily derail our best-laid plans for weight loss.

1. Learn to avoid your triggers. Eating unhealthy snacks can be a habit. Similarly, there are many regular triggers that create the feeling of hunger that are also habits. Therefore, you can weaken old cravings and the things that trigger hunger pangs by breaking these habits. It takes time to make the switch, but it can be done. If you decide to eat fruit as a snack, after a while you will start to crave fruit. If you take the back door away from the gym to avoid the snack food shop, you will get used to it. You can adapt to the feelings of temptation and after a while, you get used to them.

2. Eliminate your temptation. Simply removing tempting snack foods from your home and bypassing the sections in the shopping centers with the cake shops and snack outlets works wonders.

3. Eat a few nuts. Drink two glasses of water and eat an ounce of nuts (12 almonds, 6 walnuts or 20 peanuts). Within 15-20 minutes this will dampen your hunger cravings.

4. Eat a vitamin B tablet. If you regularly take vitamin B tablets, delay popping the pill until you feeling hungry. It suppresses the appetite.

5. Deal with your stress and anxiety without eating. Stress and anxiety are major triggers for cravings. People eat for comfort. Stress may exaggerate the feelings of being down and depressed. You need to break the habit of reaching out for a burger. It may be beneficial to learn deep breathing exercises and other ways to relieve the stress. Going for a walk or a jog works very well especially at high intensity. Eat healthy foods with low calories and fat if you must eat.

6. Avoid being tired. Cravings sneak up on you when you get tired. Take a nap and ensure you are getting enough sleep at night.

7. Use distractions as cravings are generally very short-lived. Hunger bouts and food cravings typically only last about ten minutes; simply diverting your mind onto some other activity that covers this amount of time will delay the need to eat. Ring a friend, listen to music, go for a walk, meditate or simply do something else for a while.

8. Plan to avoid temptations. Vary your usual routine to avoid going past the bakery or pizza shop. This sounds simplistic but it does work.

9. Fill up on fiber, snack on fiber. Often the hunger pangs develop more quickly if your general diet is poor, especially eating foods rich in processed carbohydrates. If you eat fiber-rich foods and bulky low-calorie foods, they will take longer to be processed and you won't feel hungry as quickly.

10. Avoid the sense of deprivation. Sometimes keeping to a diet is hard because dieters adopt feelings that they have to deprive themselves of their favorite foods, or even that they need to punish themselves. This is a recipe for failure because it is so easy to say "why should I be deprived of what I love?" Successful dieting requires a lifetime change in lifestyle and eating habits, which is not about deprivation, but developing new 'likes.'

11. Eat slow, snack on things that take a long time to eat. It takes 15-20 minutes for your body to realize "hey I'm full." So it is very easy to overshoot and eat far more than what is needed to suppress the hunger pang. So, the longer it takes to consume the food, the better. Avoid fast foods, choose 'slow' foods. Eating some celery and carrot sticks with some healthy dip takes a lot longer than downing a burger and shake, especially when you prepare the dip.

12. Stay hydrated and drink water when you feel hungry. Drink lots of water, coffee, herbal tea, soda water and other healthy low-calorie drinks as much as you can, and especially when you feel hungry. Some people eat because they are thirsty. When hunger strikes, first drink some water. Remember that a bout of hunger usually only lasts 15-20 minutes. Drinking fills your stomach for longer than this and can delay the hunger pangs.

Foods And Drinks That Kill Your Effort:

The foods you eat can have a major effect on your weight. Some foods, like full-fat yogurt, coconut oil and eggs, help with weight loss. Other foods, especially processed and refined products, can make you gain weight.

Here are foods to avoid when you're trying to lose weight.

1. French Fries and Potato Chips

Whole potatoes are healthy and filling, but french fries and potato chips are not. They are very high in calories, and it's easy to eat way too many of them. In observational studies, consuming french fries and potato chips has been linked to weight gain. One study even found that potato chips may contribute to more weight gain per serving than any other food. What's more, baked, roasted or fried potatoes may contain cancer-causing substances called acrylamides. Therefore, it's best to eat plain, boiled potatoes.

Bottom line: French fries and potato chips are unhealthy and fattening. On the other hand, whole, boiled potatoes are very healthy and help fill you up.

2. Sugary Drinks

Sugar-sweetened beverages, like soda, are some of the unhealthiest consumables on the planet. They are strongly associated with weight gain and can have disastrous health effects when consumed in excess. Even though sugary drinks contain a lot of calories, your brain doesn't register them like solid food. Liquid sugar calories don't make you feel full, and you won't eat less food to compensate. Instead, you end up adding these calories on top of your normal intake. If you are serious about losing weight, consider giving up sugary drinks altogether.

Bottom line: Sugary drinks can negatively affect your weight and general health. If weight loss is your goal, then giving up soda and similar drinks may have a significant impact.

3. White Bread

White bread is highly refined and often contains a lot of added sugar. It is high on the glycemic index and can spike your blood sugar levels. One study of 9,267 people found that eating two slices (120 grams) of white bread per day was linked to a 40% greater risk of weight gain and obesity.

Bottom line: White bread is made from very fine flour, and can spike your blood sugar levels, leading to overeating. With that being said, there are many other types of bread you can eat.

4. Candy Bars

Candy bars are extremely unhealthy. They pack a lot of added sugar, added oils, and refined flour into a small package.

Candy bars are high in calories and low in nutrients. An average-sized candy bar covered in chocolate can contain around 200–300 calories, and extra-large bars may contain even more.

Unfortunately, you can find candy bars everywhere. They are even strategically placed in stores in order to tempt consumers into buying them impulsively. If you are craving a snack, eat a piece of fruit or a handful of nuts instead.

Bottom line: Candy bars consist of unhealthy ingredients like sugar, refined flour, and added oils. They are high in calories, but not very filling.

5. Most Fruit Juices

Most fruit juices you find at the supermarket have very little in common with whole fruit. Fruit juices are highly processed and loaded with sugar. In fact, they can contain just as much sugar and calories as soda, if not more. Also, fruit juice usually has no fiber and doesn't require chewing. This means that a glass of orange juice won't have the same effects on fullness as an orange, making it easy to consume large quantities in a short amount of time.

Bottom line: Fruit juice is high in calories and added sugar, but usually contains no fiber. It is best to stick to whole fruit.

6. Pastries, Cookies and Cakes

Pastries, cookies and cakes are packed with unhealthy ingredients like added sugar and refined flour. They may also contain artificial trans fats, which are very harmful and linked to many diseases. Pastries, cookies and cakes are not very satisfying, and you will likely become hungry very quickly after eating these high-calorie, low-nutrient foods.

If you're craving something sweet, reach for a piece of dark chocolate instead.

Bottom line: Pastries, cookies and cakes often contain large amounts of added sugar, refined flour, and sometimes trans fat. These foods are high in calories, but not very filling.

7. Some Types of Alcohol (Especially Beer)

Alcohol provides more calories than carbs and protein, or about seven calories per gram. Drinking alcohol in moderation seems to be fine and is actually linked to reduced weight gain. Heavy drinking, on the other hand, is associated with increased weight gain.

Bottom Line: If you are trying to lose weight, you may want to consider cutting back on alcohol or skipping it altogether. Wine in small amounts seems to be fine.

8. Ice Cream

Ice cream is incredibly delicious but very unhealthy. It is high in calories, and most types are loaded with sugar. A small portion of ice cream is fine every now and then, but the problem is that it's very easy to consume massive amounts in one sitting. Consider making your own ice cream, using less sugar and healthier ingredients like full-fat yogurt and fruit.

Also, serve yourself a small portion and put the ice cream away so that you won't end up eating too much.

Bottom Line: Store-bought ice cream is high in sugar, and homemade ice cream is a better alternative. Remember to be mindful of portions, as it's very easy to eat too much ice cream.

9. Pizza

Pizza is a very popular fast food. However, commercially made pizzas also happen to be very unhealthy. Homemade pizza sauce is also healthier, since supermarket varieties can contain lots of sugar. Another option is to look for a pizza place that makes healthier pizzas. Yes, they're out there.

Bottom Line: Commercial pizzas are often made from highly refined and processed ingredients. A homemade pizza with healthier ingredients is a much better option.

10. High-Calorie Coffee Drinks

Coffee contains several biologically active substances, most importantly caffeine. These chemicals can boost your metabolism and increase fat burning, at least in the short term.

However, the adverse effects of adding unhealthy ingredients like artificial cream and sugar outweigh these positive results. High-calorie coffee drinks are no better than soda. They're loaded with empty calories that can equal a whole meal.

If you like coffee, it's best to stick to plain, black coffee when trying to lose weight. Adding a little cream or milk is fine too. Just avoid adding sugar, high-calorie creamers and other unhealthy ingredients.

Bottom Line: Plain, black coffee can be very healthy and even help you burn fat. However, high-calorie coffee drinks that contain artificial ingredients are very unhealthy and fattening.

11. Foods High in Added Sugar

Added sugar is probably the worst thing in the modern diet. Excess amounts have been linked to some of the most serious diseases in the world today. Foods high in added sugar usually provide tons of empty calories, but are not very filling. Examples of foods that may contain massive amounts of added sugar include sugary breakfast cereals, granola bars and low-fat, flavored yogurt.

You should be especially careful when selecting "low-fat" or "fat-free" foods, as manufacturers often add lots of sugar to make up for the flavor that's lost when the fat is removed.

Bottom line: Added sugar is one of the unhealthiest ingredients in the modern diet. Many products, such as low-fat and fat-free foods, seem healthy but are loaded with sugar.

Take Home Message

The worst foods for weight loss are highly processed junk foods. These foods are typically loaded with added sugar, refined wheat and/or added fats.

If you're not sure if a food is healthy or unhealthy, read the label.

However, watch out for the different names for sugar and misleading health claims.

Also, remember to consider the serving sizes. Some healthy foods, like nuts, dried fruit and cheese, are high in calories, and it can be very easy to eat too much.

The Importance of Cardio Workouts

Do cardio workouts for maximum weight loss and be amazed by the overall results. This workout type is specifically aimed at flexing and strengthening the heart muscles by encouraging a boost in heart rate in a healthy way. Cardio workouts additionally assist in improving blood flow, burn calories and oxygenate tissue cells and blood. Establishing great cardiovascular structure is essential for overall health and wellbeing. The primary factor in continued efficiency is to identify methods to better cardio exercises gradually, thus accomplishing maximum weight loss.

Indeed, there are several kinds of cardio exercises and combinations of workouts with which numerous individuals are familiar. But, what is important about any exercise regime or fitness activity is that you ought to constantly make a choice that will fulfill your needs best. The type of workout you choose will be based considerably on your physical capability. Before starting any exercise routine, have a health check up or physical and also seek the advice of a medical practitioner or fitness personnel who's able to assist you in finding activities and programs that are perfect for you.

1. Maximize Your Endurance

Try your best to be consistent with your routine. Working out for 30 minutes for three days each week, over a six-week period is a good start. This would be manageable for most people. As one's body adapts to this activity, slowly increase your maximum time by about five minutes each week in order to progressively boost stamina. Never push your body too rigorously, because you don't want to wind up injuring yourself. Try to increase workout durations each week by about 10% if possible. Take short breaks after each routine and avoid exercising for over one hour at a time.

2. Try Not To Be Bored

You are now aware that a small part of your day will be spent doing cardio exercises. In order to obtain the most from it, it is important to make sure that your mind is focused. Find a suitable method of motivating yourself to exercise. If you decide to walk, run, hike or jog, listening to music is a wonderful way for staying focused as time passes. It doesn't matter what sort of songs you play, as long as it is a selection of songs that you enjoy. Music will additionally help to relax your mind, hence reducing stress and anxiety.

Another excellent approach to maintaining interest in your workout is to perform activities that you really love. If you are into cycling, hiking, swimming, or playing sports, perform these types of activities. In all probability, you can expect to be better at things that you enjoy without much motivation. It's important to understand that your mind has supreme power over your body, and when you lose interest or cannot maintain focus, you will find it very difficult to do cardio workouts for maximum weight loss.

3. Maximize Fat Loss

For maximum fat loss during the course of cardiovascular workouts, consume a light meal around 30 minutes prior to working out. Also, avoid eating for at least an hour after exercising. This will enable your body to utilize retained fat for energy as well as burn up more calories. The result is continued fat loss as your metabolism continues to function at a high rate. One's body will likely continue burning calories after an hour of exercise. Therefore, abstain from feeding your body with extra energy for as much as one hour after a cardio workout.

4. Make Use of Your Whole Body

The amount of time that you are able to invest in cardio exercises should be spent utilizing your entire body. For instance, rather than using a fitness bike, utilize a treadmill, a tread climber or an elliptical instead. If not, do some high-impact workouts instead. Doing this will not only help to improve your overall fitness, but also burn maximum calories, work your muscles and stimulate inactive fat stores. When you use your entire body during a workout, you can potentially burn well over 100 calories more every hour than you would have normally. Great ways to use most of your body and work hard-to-reach muscles are by using a stability ball or some form of resistance equipment on your hands or feet. Use these tools to aid in the toning of your muscles and the strengthening of your arms, legs, and core.

5. Increase Your Heart Rate

Every person has a maximum pulse rate that can be reached when working out that will help to maximize weight loss. Your maximum pulse rate should be 220 minus your age. Hence, if you are currently 20 years old, your maximum heart rate will be 200 beats per minute. As you become older, your max heart rate will decrease. You should aim to do a sufficient amount of exercise to bring your heart rate to approximately 75 percent of its maximum.

Never be hesitant to attempt a wide range of exercises. Do as many 1-minute varieties as possible. This will help to maximize weight loss and prevent boredom. When you find a routine that you enjoy, stick to it, but try to implement variations. Jumping, squatting, lifting, and running are great ways to get maximum cardio efficiency for weight loss. Add a mixture of these activities to your exercise routine.

The process of losing weight during cardio exercises happens over a prolonged period and can prove to be difficult initially. Nevertheless, while you advance in your exercise program, your body will eventually adapt. Try to make your cardiovascular exercises as efficient and effective as possible. This will certainly not just greatly enhance its impact, but additionally help you lose weight and maintain a healthy body.

How to Keep The Weight Off After Losing It

If you have worked hard to lose weight, you will want to enjoy your new healthy weight for the rest of your life. Here are ten tips for achieving lifelong weight maintenance.

1. Monitor Your Weight

Weigh yourself once a week (do not weigh yourself too often as it is natural for your weight to fluctuate daily). Use your bathroom scales, or find a pair of pants that are comfortable at your goal weight and identify if they get significantly tighter or looser.

You should set an upper and a lower limit on your weight (a Dietitian can help you set appropriate limits). If you hit your upper or lower limit, seek professional help from a Dietitian as soon as possible. DO NOT procrastinate for too long—it is much easier to reverse a 1-2lb weight gain than it is to reverse a 5-7lb weight gain!

2. Monitor Your Eating Patterns

It is important that you maintain a consistent eating pattern for the rest of your life - do not change it too drastically on weekends or when you go away for holidays.

Documenting what you eat is a great habit. By keeping a food diary, you can ensure that you are eating the right amounts of food from each of the five food groups and check that you are eating regularly (that means not skipping any meals).

3. Exercise

To maintain your weight, you need to exercise at a moderate intensity (a rate at which your heart rate is elevated but you can still carry out a conversation) for at least 150 minutes per week. A great way to achieve this is to walk for 30 minutes on five days of every week. For the fitter members of the audience, you can try vigorous cardiovascular exercise such as jogging for 20 minutes a day on three days of every week.

4. Continue to Set Goals

The goal of weight loss is change, whereas the goal of weight maintenance is no change. It can be harder to eat well and exercise when you do not see results for the effort you are putting in. To account for this, try setting other life goals that are better enjoyed at a lower weight (e.g. joining a community fun walk or going traveling).

5. Reward Yourself

When you were losing weight, you were probably enjoying the associated rewards such as the compliments from other people, the excitement of fitting into smaller clothes and the joy of jumping onto the scales and seeing a smaller number. Therefore, you will need a new set of rewards for maintaining your weight. Perhaps you can treat yourself to a massage, buy a book or have a manicure or a pedicure at the end of every month. Continue these rewards for at least the first few years after weight loss.

6. Enlist Support

While you were losing weight, you probably received encouragement from family, friends and health professionals. Weight maintenance can be just as difficult as weight loss at times - and it can be a more isolated process. However, it does not have to be that way. Tell the important people in your life that maintaining your healthy weight is important to you, and that you would like their support and encouragement for the long term.

7. Remain Vigilant

It is easy to get complacent when you achieve your weight loss goal. People sometimes fall into the trap of thinking, "I can have that extra scoop of chocolate ice cream for dessert because I have lost a lot of weight and I am feeling really good." Just because you have lost weight, doesn't mean that extra calories don't add up anymore.

It is important to treat yourself from time to time, but it is also important to recognize when extra treats are creeping into your diet too often. By keeping a food diary (or just listing the extras you are having on a notepad) you can identify how frequently you are treating yourself. You should consume no more than 2-3 treats per week, and whenever you consume a treat limit yourself to a 200-Calorie portion.

8. Be Organized

It is hard to manage your weight when the rest of your life is in chaos. Leave plenty of time for relaxation, sleeping, shopping for healthy foods, preparing healthy meals and exercising.

9. Maintain your Self Esteem

Maintain a good level of self-esteem—do not link how you feel about yourself to your weight. Be happy with your weight and proud of the weight loss that you have achieved.

10. Do Not Use Food to Stabilize Your Moods

If you are feeling stressed or upset, find a non-food related way of calming yourself - go for a walk, take a bath or call a friend.

Lastly, do not forget that weight maintenance can be just as challenging as weight loss (if not more so in the first two years). Understand that it gets easier with time, and by following this advice you will be well on your way to success

Myths About Dieting and Workouts

There are many unhealthy misconceptions about weight loss. One needs to be aware of actual facts and faulty information. This information has the power to make your journey more effective. Wrong facts take a toll on your health and goals. Thus, it's better to educate yourself correctly about various factors that contribute to weight loss and healthy eating.

1. Diets don't work. If you eat less calories, you will lose weight. It is not normally the diet that does not work but the restrictions a diet creates. If you chose a diet that introduces a healthier lifestyle but still allows you some treats, you are more likely to succeed in losing weight.

2. The heavier you are, the more calories you need to burn everyday. Actually, it is the reverse. You can have more calories and lose weight as your body must work extra hard to move the excess weight around, conequently burning more calories. However, as you lose weight, you will have to drop your calorie intake accordingly.

3. Being overweight is in my genes. Scientists have been hard at work trying to identify if there is a 'fat' gene and have seen that there is - but only in a microscopic population of the world. More than the gene, those who are obese have normally inherited the eating and exercise habits of their parents and it is this that leads to weight gain.

4. Eating after six o'clock will make you gain weight as you don't burn it off. Eating in the evening will not make you gain weight. In fact, many people get hungry around dinner time and it is natural for your body to ask for food. What will pile on the pounds is the type of food you have for dinner/supper - avoid sweet treats such as cakes and biscuits or those high in fat.

5. All carbohydrates are bad. Carbs have had a difficult time recently with the Atkins Diet becoming so popular, but they don't actually deserve the bad press they get. Whilst a high carbohydrate diet (potatoes, bread, rice, pasta etc.) will not actually make you gain weight, it is the fat added to the carbohydrates in the sauces and cooking methods that will raise your calorie count.

6. Dairy products are fattening. Dairy products are very good for you as they are packed full of vitamins and minerals that your body needs to stay healthy. Many women are now beginning to suffer from osteoarthritis as a result of restricting dairy products (milk, cheese, yogurt etc.) from their diet. There are loads of low-fat dairy products on the market these days; you will not have to give up the calcium content or taste by trying them. Indeed, semi-skimmed and skimmed milk has slightly more calcium than full fat.

7. Wheat intolerance causes my weight gain. Wheat intolerance is very popular these days and often takes the blame for weight gain. However, there are very few of us (less than 0.1%) that actually suffer from this condition. People who have a wheat-free diet may very well lose weight, but this is normally because they cut things such as pizza, cakes, biscuits, puddings and processed foods.

8. Low-fat foods are the best way to help you lose weight. Just because something is marked 'low-fat' or 'fat-free' does not necessarily mean that it has less calories than full-fat items. In fact, some may even have more calories as they have extra additives such as sugars and thickeners to help improve the taste and texture. People also think they can have more of something if it is marked as low fat, but this is rarely true.

9. Anything marked 'healthy eating' is the best for helping you lose weight. Whilst most 'healthy eating' ranges cut out on the fat content, they pay little attention to the salt, calorie or sugar content. Also, many 'healthy eating' ranges actually offer smaller portions meaning you reach for that high-calorie snack as soon as the hunger pangs kick in.

10. Frozen or canned food is not as good as fresh food. In actuality, frozen or canned food can have a higher vitamin content than fresh food. Most frozen food is frozen at around two hours after picking; the same applies to canning. This means there is very little vitamin loss as compared to fresh fruits and vegetables that may take days to get onto the store shelves. Make sure you opt for fruit that is canned in juice rather than syrup and avoid salted vegetables.

11. Cereal bars are much better for you than a chocolate bar. While the health virtues of wheat, oats and whole grains in cereal bars cannot be denied, most also contain sugars, honey, glucose or the like and can have a higher calorie content than a small bar of chocolate. Even dark chocolate has its own health virtues—in moderation.

12. Vegetarian diets are the best for losing weight. Whilst a vegetarian diet is great for meeting your five a day quota, they can also be packed with high-calorie foods.

13. The best option is salad when eating out. Salad is great for weight loss, as well as making up a five a day portion, but can actually be higher in fat than steak and chips. Salad served with dressing, croutons, bacon bits, cheese, mayonnaise or dressings can be extremely high in fat, calorie and salt content with little vitamin or mineral benefit. If you are choosing a salad, make sure it is a plain option without dressing.

14. Organic foods are better for you than non-organic. Whilst it is true that organic farming methods are better for the environment as well as reducing chemicals in your fruit and vegetables, eating them does not mean you will reduce your calorie count. Organic foods such as cakes, biscuits and puddings are equally as high in calorie content.

15. All nuts are fattening and must be avoided during dieting. Nuts are high in fat, but not saturated fats. They actually contain heart-healthy monounsaturated fat as well as fiber, vitamins and minerals. Even better, research has shown that a diet that contains a small amount of fat—including peanuts and peanut butter—can help lose weight as well as maintaining a healthy heart.

16. Frozen fruits and vegetables are less nutritious. It is always best to eat fresh fruits and vegetables for a healthy diet. Understandably, it is not always possible to have access to fresh produce. In this scenario, the next best option surely goes to frozen fruits and vegetables. Fruits and veggies when frozen retain most of their nutrients and lie close to fresh produce for health benefits. Just make sure there is no salt, sugar or preservatives added and they are good to go for.

17. Skipping meals will help you lose weight. Skipping meals is not at all healthy if you are up for weight loss or not. Especially if you are exercising, it is the worst thing you can do for your body. Depriving your body of essential nutrients can lead to a weak immune system and fatigue which will show visible signs in the long run.

Another problem with skipping meals is it will eventually lead to food cravings high in sugar and fat which overall defeat the purpose of your weight loss big time. Instead of skipping meals, you should be vigilant in keeping yourself full with a healthy and balanced diet (as suggested by a dietitian).

18. Carbohydrates are bad for weight loss. Carbohydrates are actually a great source of energy. The body uses carbs as fuel to burn body fat during workouts. You can make it a point to avoid processed carbs and select healthy carb options for your meals or snacks. Complex carbs provide continuous energy over a long period of time and come from foods like whole grains, beans or nuts. Simple carbs give short spikes of energy and are found in foods like bread, sugar, cereal, etc.

19. Early morning is the best time for a workout. You will get same results irrespective of your workout timings. What is more important is to work out regularly. However, early morning is good to do breathing exercises to bring in more fresh oxygen into your body that will keep you fresh and energized all day long. Morning is a good time to work out as your mind is free of all day stimulations and activities, so you focus more on your workout than other things.

However, if you are unable to workout in mornings for any reasons, do not be hesitant from doing it at another time during the day. Just keep moving your body around even if not in the mornings or same time of the day.

Your genes decide your metabolic rate and body weight. Genes passed on to you by your parents do play their role in weight loss. Though, they do not completely control how you lose weight. Just working around your body, taking into account how genes make your body function can lead you to your dream body. This is the reason why particular things work for some people and not others. Your body tries to keep your weight within a specific range, called your set point. This range is greatly influenced by your genetic makeup. However, your actual weight within that range is influenced by your lifestyle or environment. So, let genes do their work and you do yours.

20. It is best to starve before an event. When you starve on food, you are not only depriving yourself of essential nutrients that are required to provide you energy and a healthy glow, but also sending the wrong signal to your mind which ultimately leads to your body storing food as fat for future use. What you are doing is storing fat and setting yourself up for a bloated face, as well as other parts of your body. Instead, try increasing your physical activity in any form. If you want to avoid sugar and sweets, stick with healthy and balanced diets.

21. You can cut out all the fats. It's only natural to associate cutting all the fat out of your diet/eating habits with losing weight or assisting in reaching your desired weight/goal. It seems logical and sounds like it makes a lot of sense. The only bad part about this "wonderful idea" is that all your body's major organs require fats in order to function correctly and efficiently. Your brain being one of the most important benefactors of fats along with your muscles and all other major body organs. What is not needed is the obscene level of carbohydrates you have been consuming over an extended period of time in an attempt to get muscled up.

Remember, no matter who you are or what weight class you are in, believe in yourself and understand that anything is possible with the right amount of effort and dedication. There is room for all of us to improve our physical appearance, but don't let that limit you from living your life on your own terms. Stay confident, stay consistent, and always remember to eat smart, not less.

** Thank you very much for sharing an interest in my book. As a writer, I work hard to create and bring accurate, relative content to my readers. If you enjoyed this book, please leave a review on Amazon. If you have any questions, concerns, or criticism, please feel free to email me directly at kconnorsbooks@gmail.com. **

Printed in Great Britain
by Amazon